My First Time

Getting Glasses

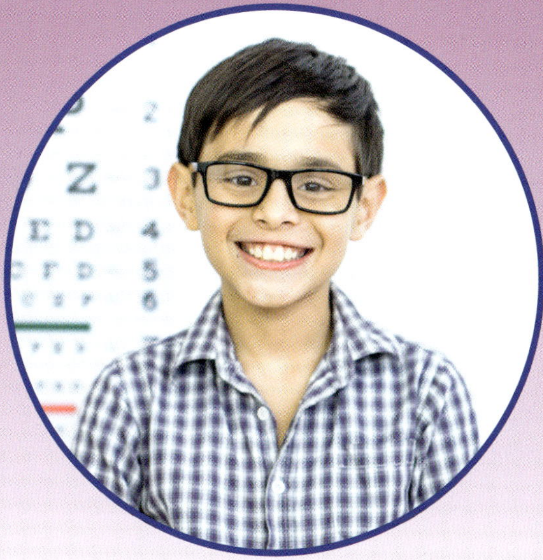

by Jeri Cipriano

LOOK! BOOKS™

Red Chair Press Egremont, Massachusetts

Look! Books are produced and published by Red Chair Press:
Red Chair Press LLC PO Box 333 South Egremont, MA 01258-0333

FREE Educator Guides at www.redchairpress.com/free-resources

Publisher's Cataloging-In-Publication Data

Names: Cipriano, Jeri, author.

Title: Getting glasses / by Jeri Cipriano.

Description: Egremont, Massachusetts : Red Chair Press, [2021] | Series: Look! books. My first time | Includes index and a list of resources for further reading. | Interest age level: 005-008. | Summary: "Four-eyes! Nerd! These are just some of the mean things people say to kids with glasses. But did you know some of the smartest people to ever have lived all wore glasses? Glasses help many people read better and see far-away things better. Glasses can be a secret tool to being cool"--Provided by publisher.

Identifiers: ISBN 9781643710945 (RLB hardcover) | ISBN 9781643711003 (softcover) | ISBN 9781643711065 (ebook)

Subjects: LCSH: Eyeglasses--Juvenile literature. | Eye--Care and hygiene--Juvenile literature. | Vision--Juvenile literature. | CYAC: Eyeglasses. | Eye--Care and hygiene. | Vision.

Classification: LCC RE976 .C56 2021 (print) | LCC RE976 (ebook) | DDC 617.7/522--dc23

LCCN: 2020948761

Photo credits: iStock

Printed in United States of America
0421 1P CGF21

Table of Contents

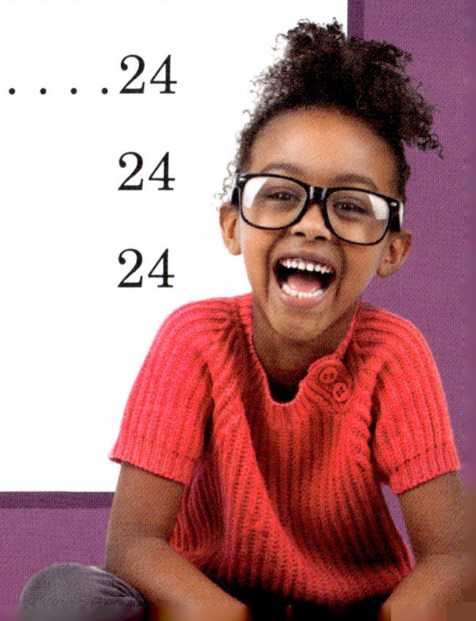

How We See

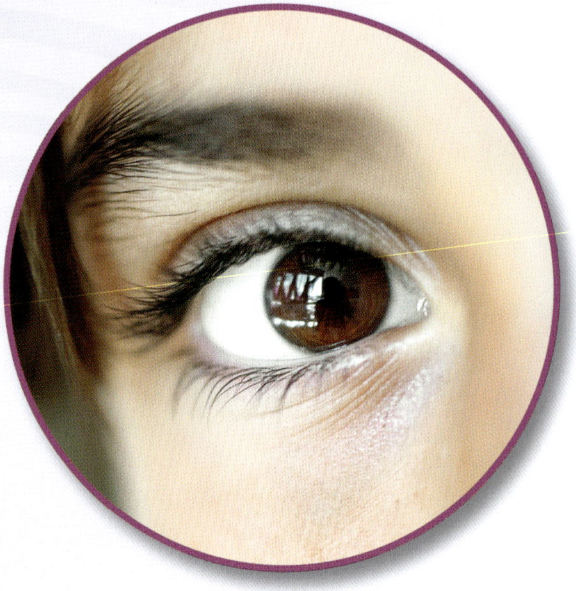

From the moment you wake up until you go to sleep, your eyes are working. There are many muscles in your body. But the muscles that control your eyes are the busiest.

Good to Know

It's almost impossible to sneeze with your eyes open.

Look Around

Your eyes take pictures of the world around you. They send these "pictures" to your brain. Your brain works out what your eyes are seeing.

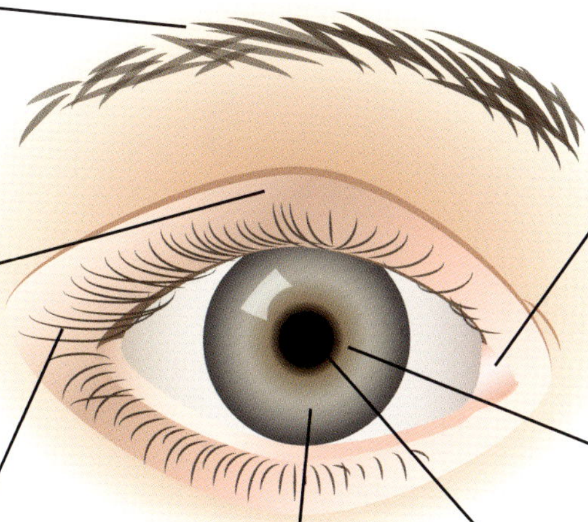

Eyebrows
keep dust and sweat from running into the eyes.

Eyelids
shut out light so you can sleep. Blink to keep eyes clean and wet with tears.

Eyelashes
catch and trap dust as eyelids close.

Cornea
is the thin clear part that covers each eye.

Tear duct
is the place where tears come from.

Iris
is the colored part of the eye.

Pupil
is the dark center that lets in light.

How Eyes Work

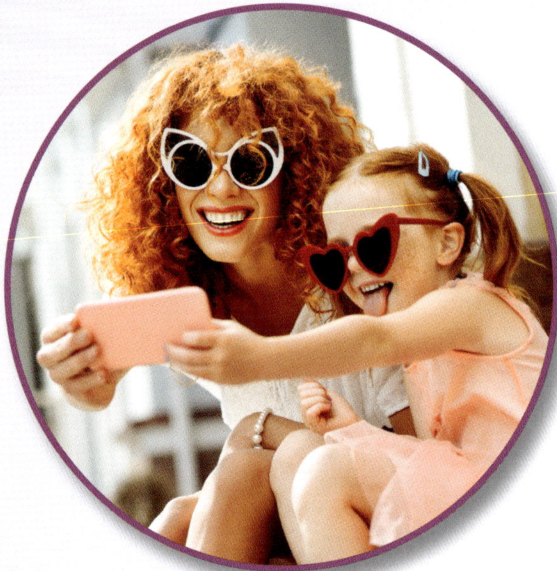

Your eyes work the way a **camera** works. Light rays from something you are looking at pass through the lens of your eye to the **retina** at the back of the eye. From there, the picture goes to the brain. Your brain sends the correct picture for you to see.

Your Brain Helps You See?

Notice how your eyes first see the **image**. It is upside down. When your eye sends the picture to your brain, your brain turns the picture the right way up for you to see.

Good to Know

Your eyes use 65% of your brain power to see. That's more than any other part of your body uses your brain.

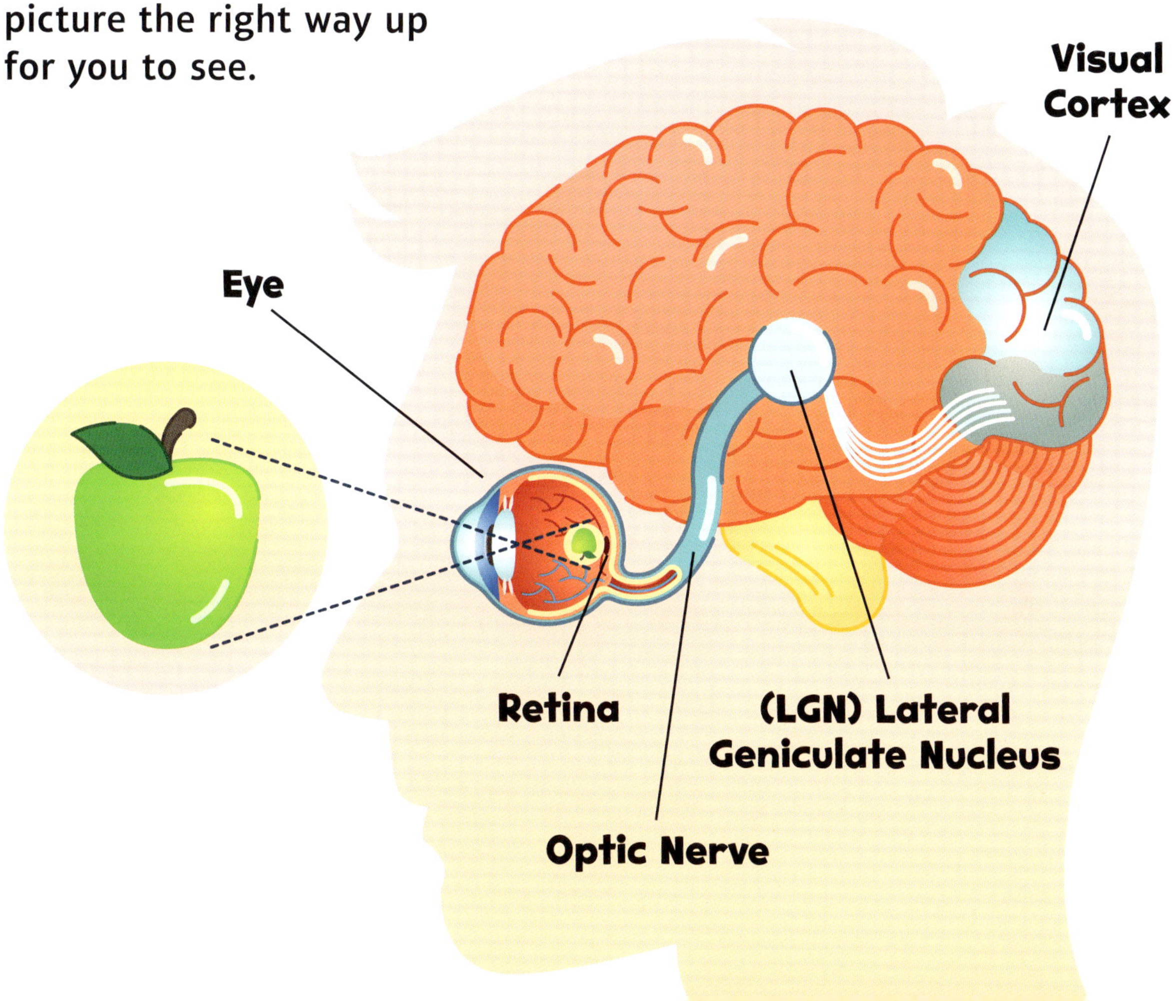

Caring for Your Eyes

Your eyes are very important. That is why you should have a check-up with an eye doctor. The doctor will make sure your eyes are healthy. Eye doctors make sure you can see clearly.

Good to Know

Your fingerprint has 40 features that make it yours alone. But the iris of your eye has 256 features! That is why eye scans are often used for security purposes.

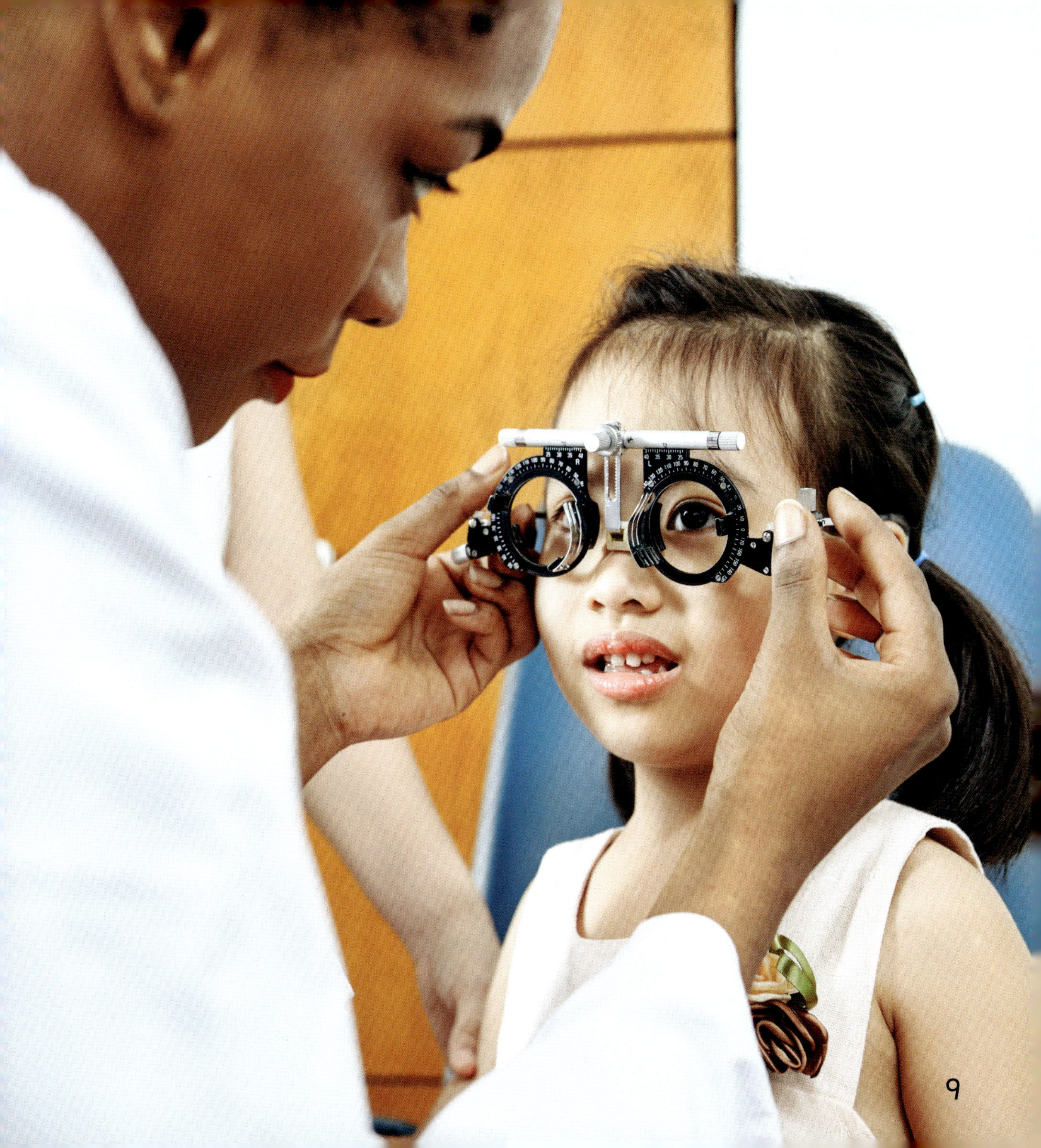

The Office Visit

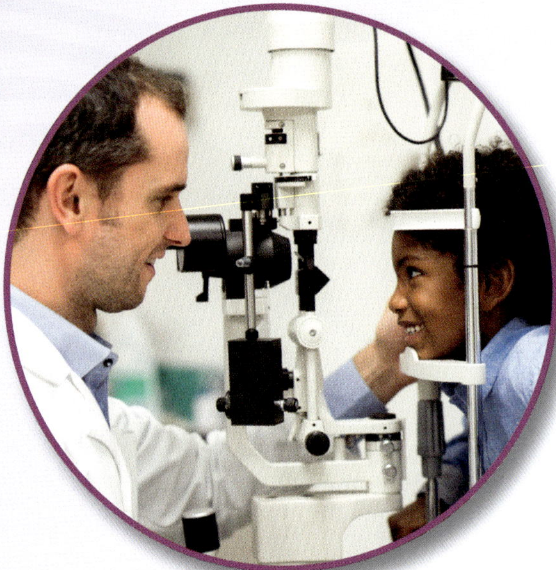

First, you will meet the doctor's helper. That person will take pictures and measurements of your eye. You rest your chin on a machine that does all the work.

Good to Know

The human eye sees only three colors: red, blue, and green. All other colors are combinations of these.

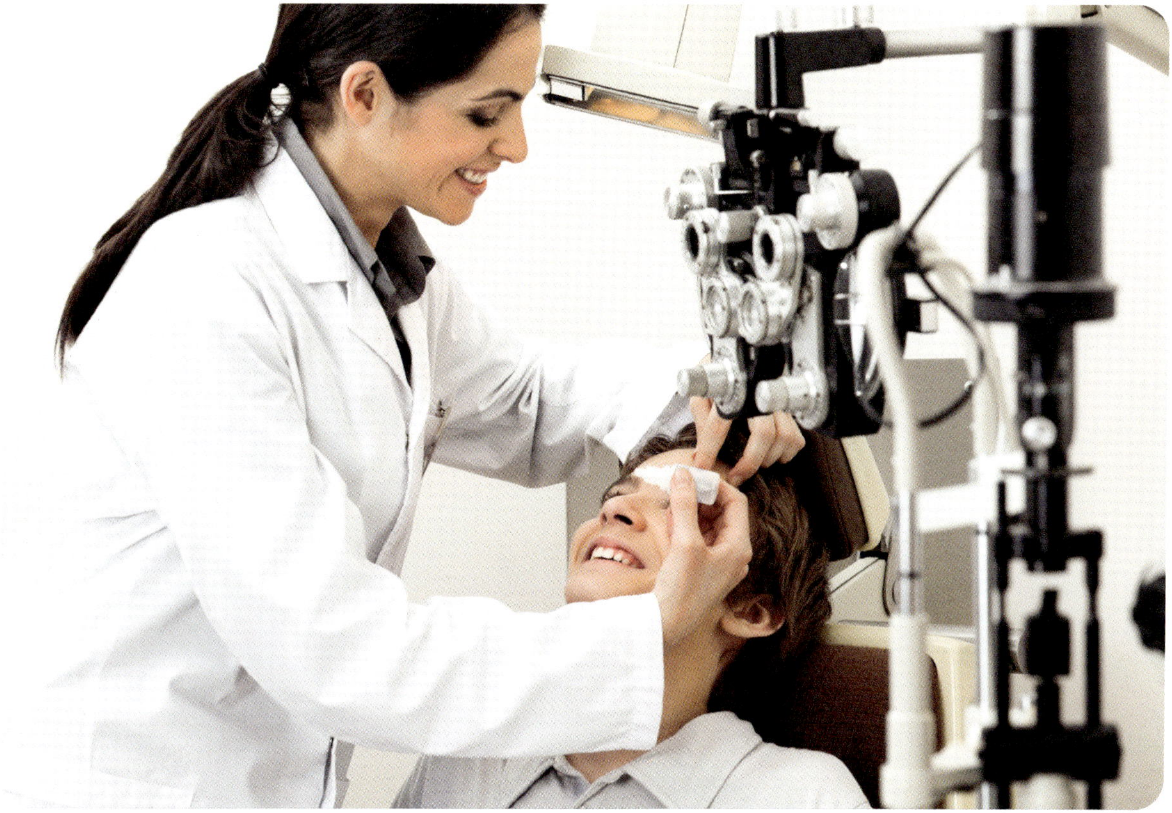

The eye doctor puts drops in your eyes. The drops let the doctor look deeply in your eyes to make sure they are healthy.

The eye doctor will ask you to read something on a paper. Then the doctor will put something on the wall to see. You will say what you see at the top—and work your way down each row.

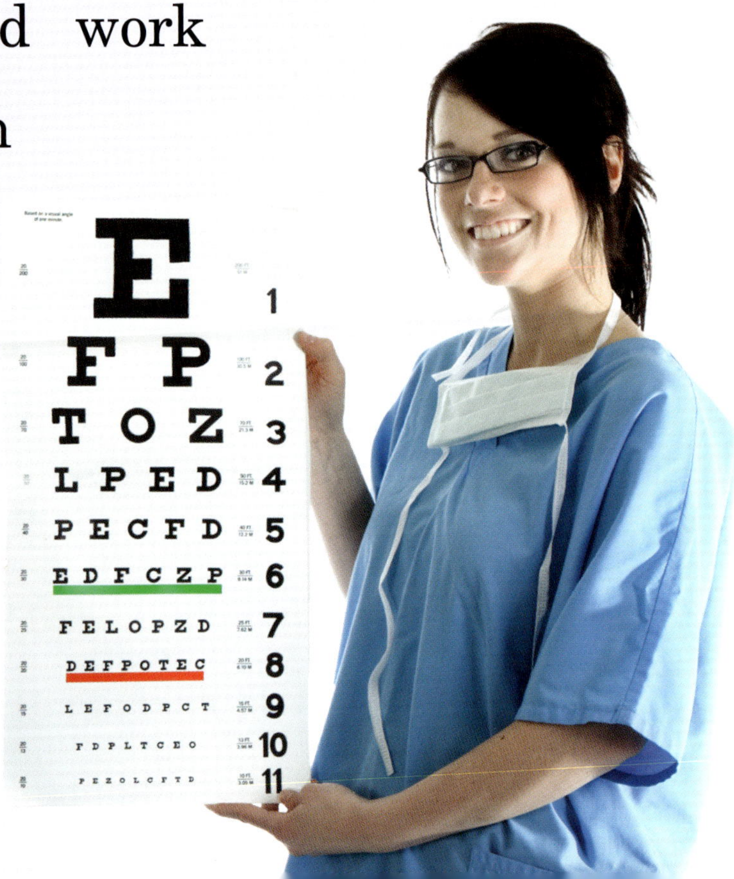

This is an example of a chart you might see.

Good to Know

Most of what we know we learn through our eyes.

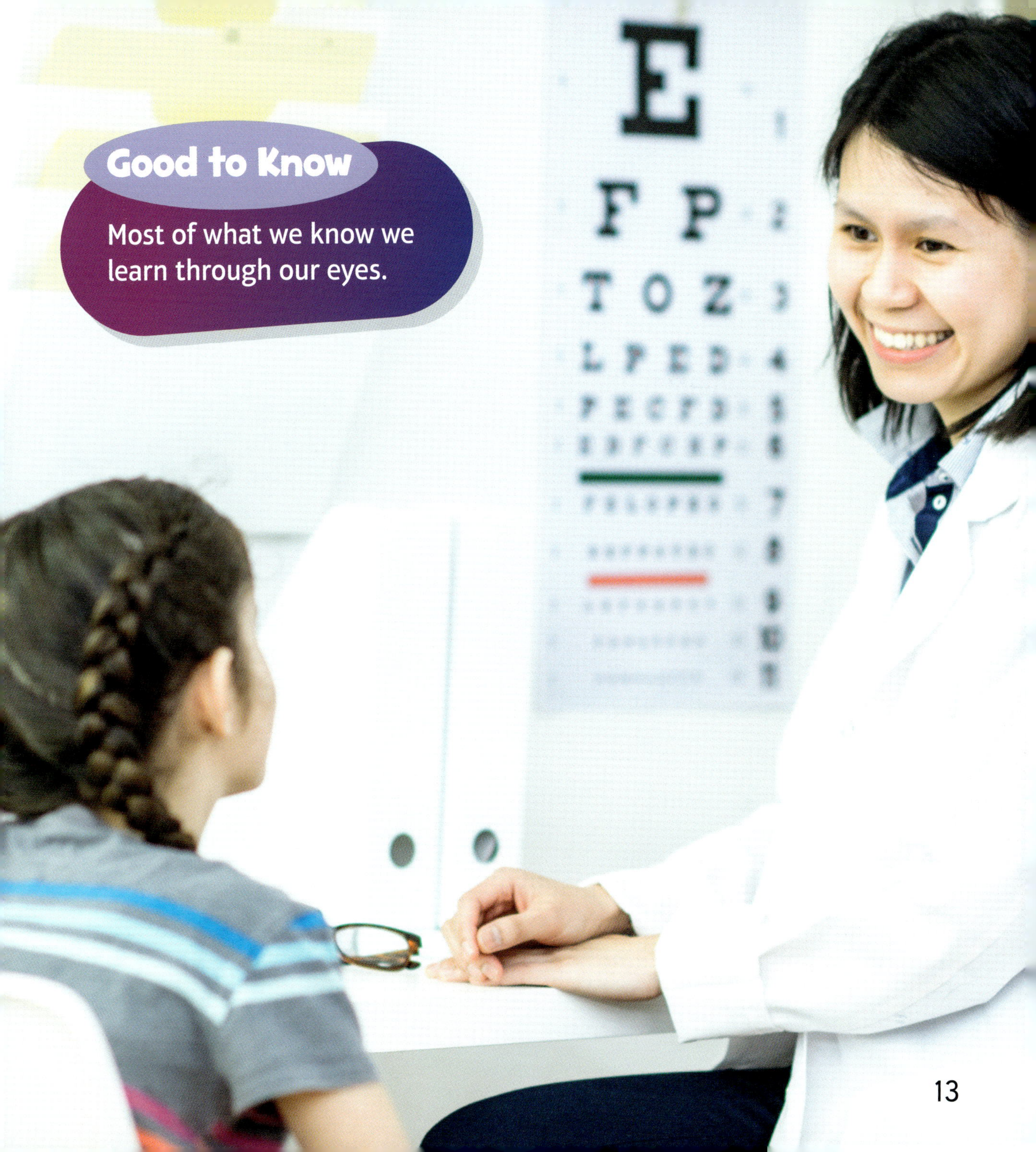

Need Glasses?

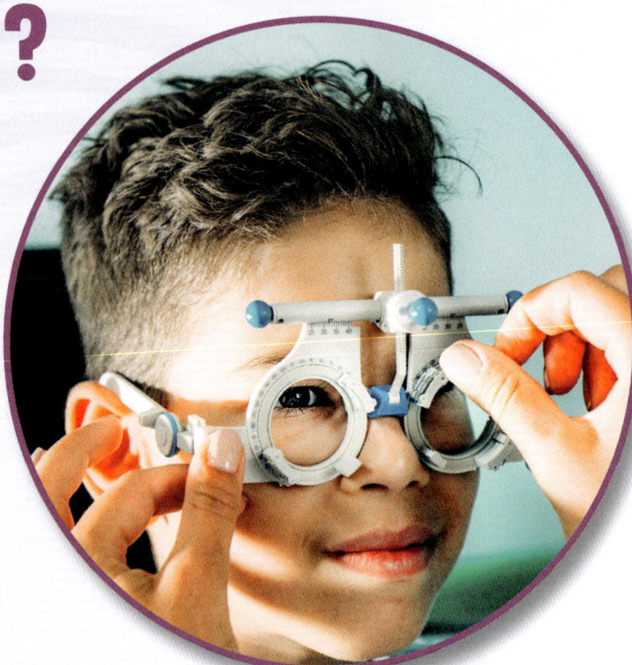

If a picture or letter is blurry, it may mean that you need glasses.

The doctor will put different lenses in front of you. You will answer questions like, “Is this better?” “What about this?”

The doctor will write down information you need to get glasses. Then the fun part comes next!

Framed!

You will visit a store that has frames for you to try on. Which frame on the faces below do you like best?

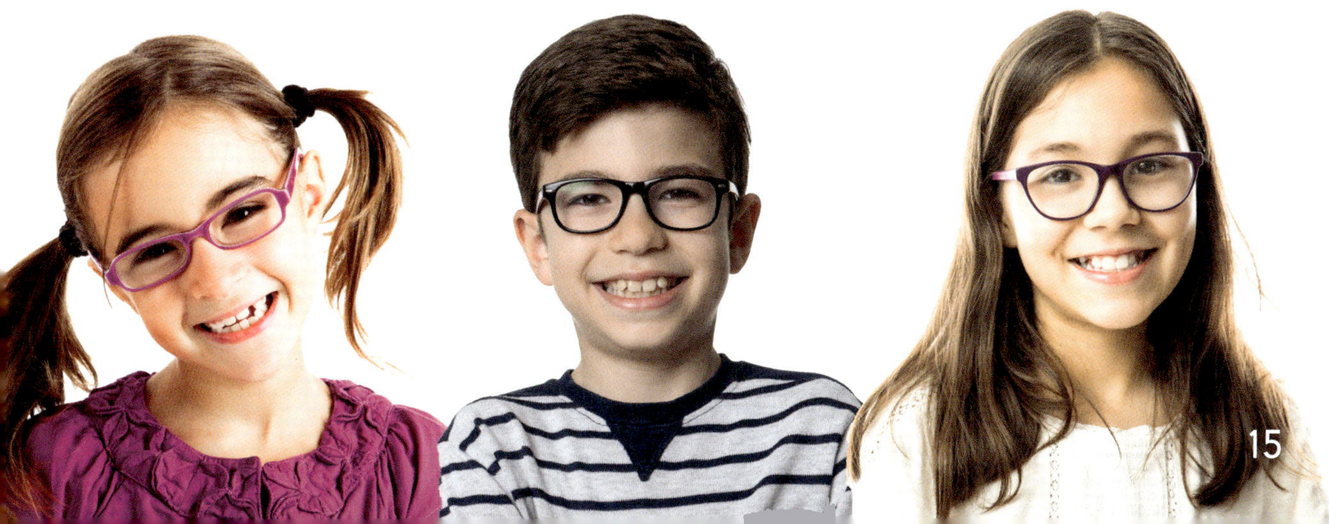

Here's Looking at You!

It's fun to choose the frames for your new glasses. You will pick your favorite color, size, and shape.

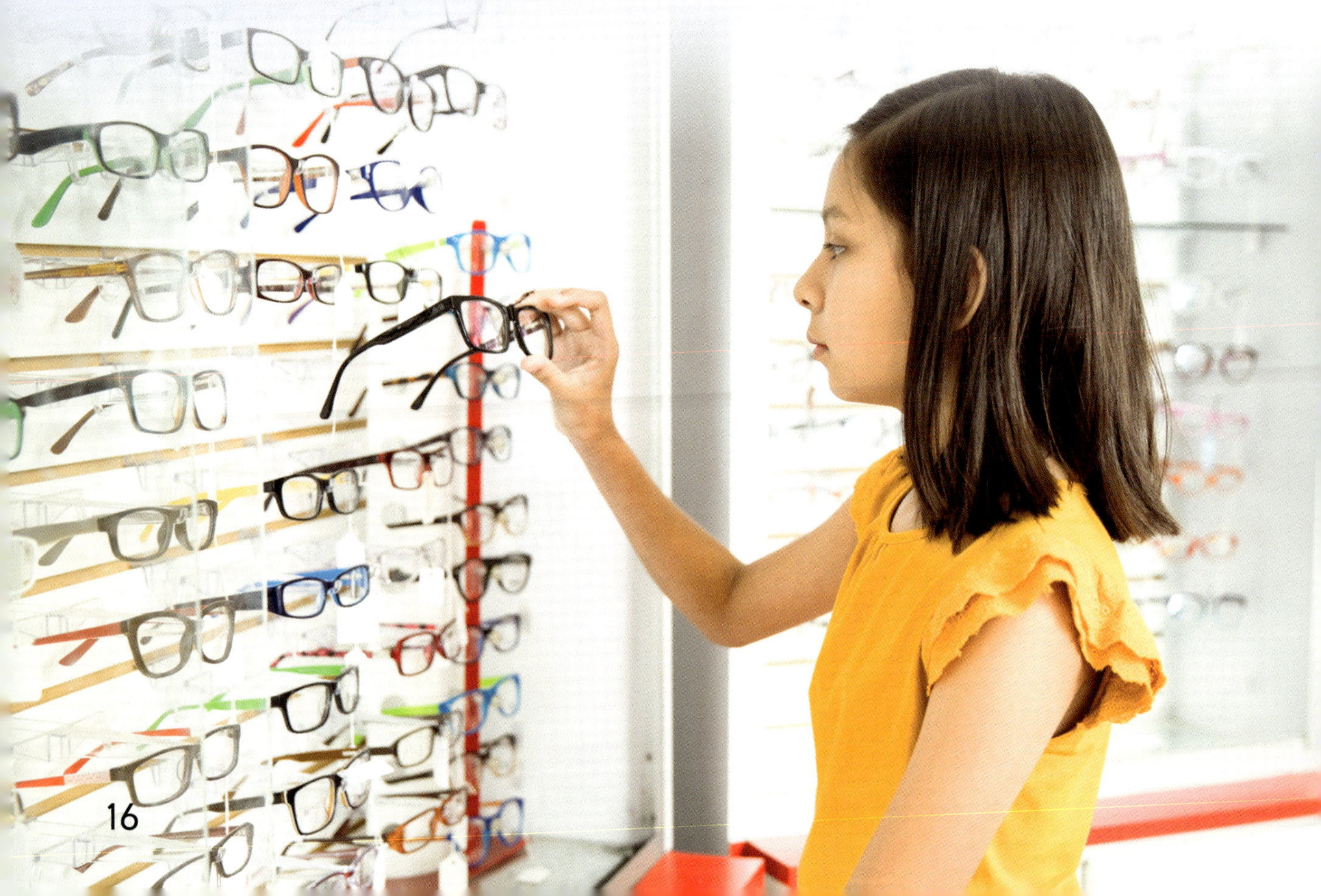

On the Face or In the Case

Give your glasses a morning wipe-down before school. Spray your glasses with a cleaner and wipe them with a soft cloth. Put your glasses in their case at night to protect them.

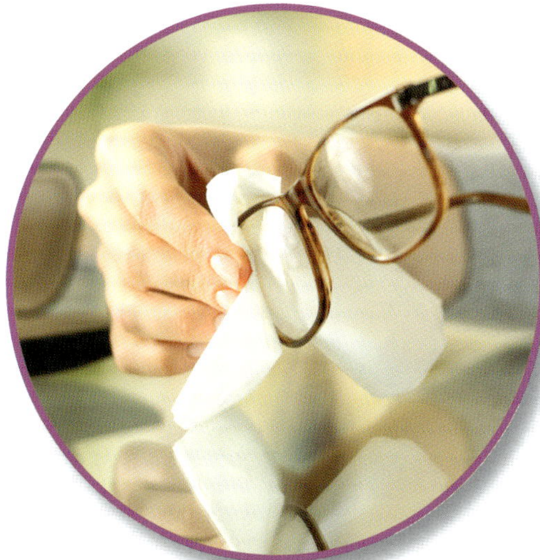

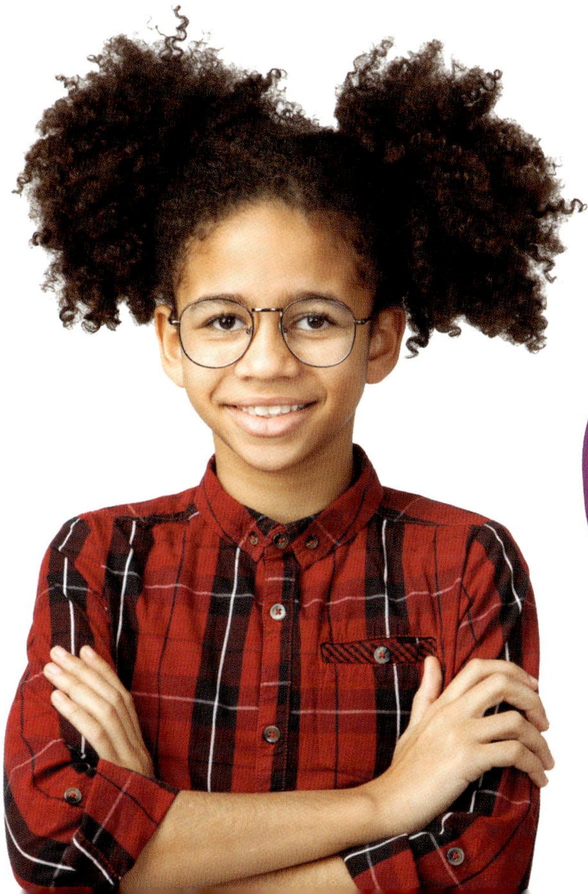

Good to Know

Your eyes have the fastest muscles in your body. That's why we say "in the blink of an eye" when something happens quickly.

Protect Your Eyes

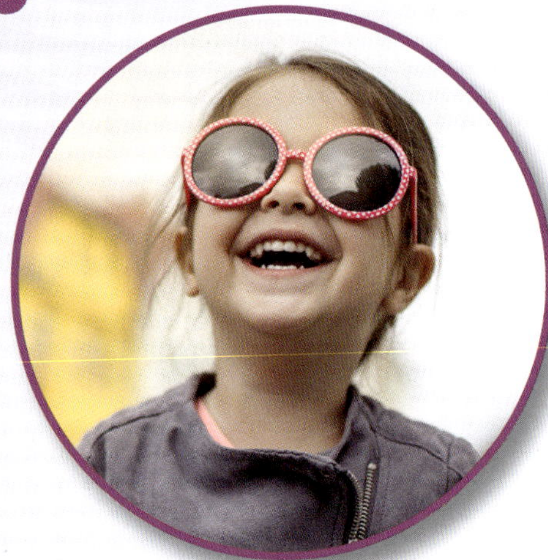

Humans' eyes can get sunburned. That is why it is important to wear sunglasses on sunny days.

Sunglasses were invented in 1929. These glasses keep harmful rays from reaching your eyes.

Good to Know

Sunglasses became popular in the 1930s. Movie stars began wearing them. Pictures of these stars appeared in magazines. Soon, all people started wearing sunglasses.

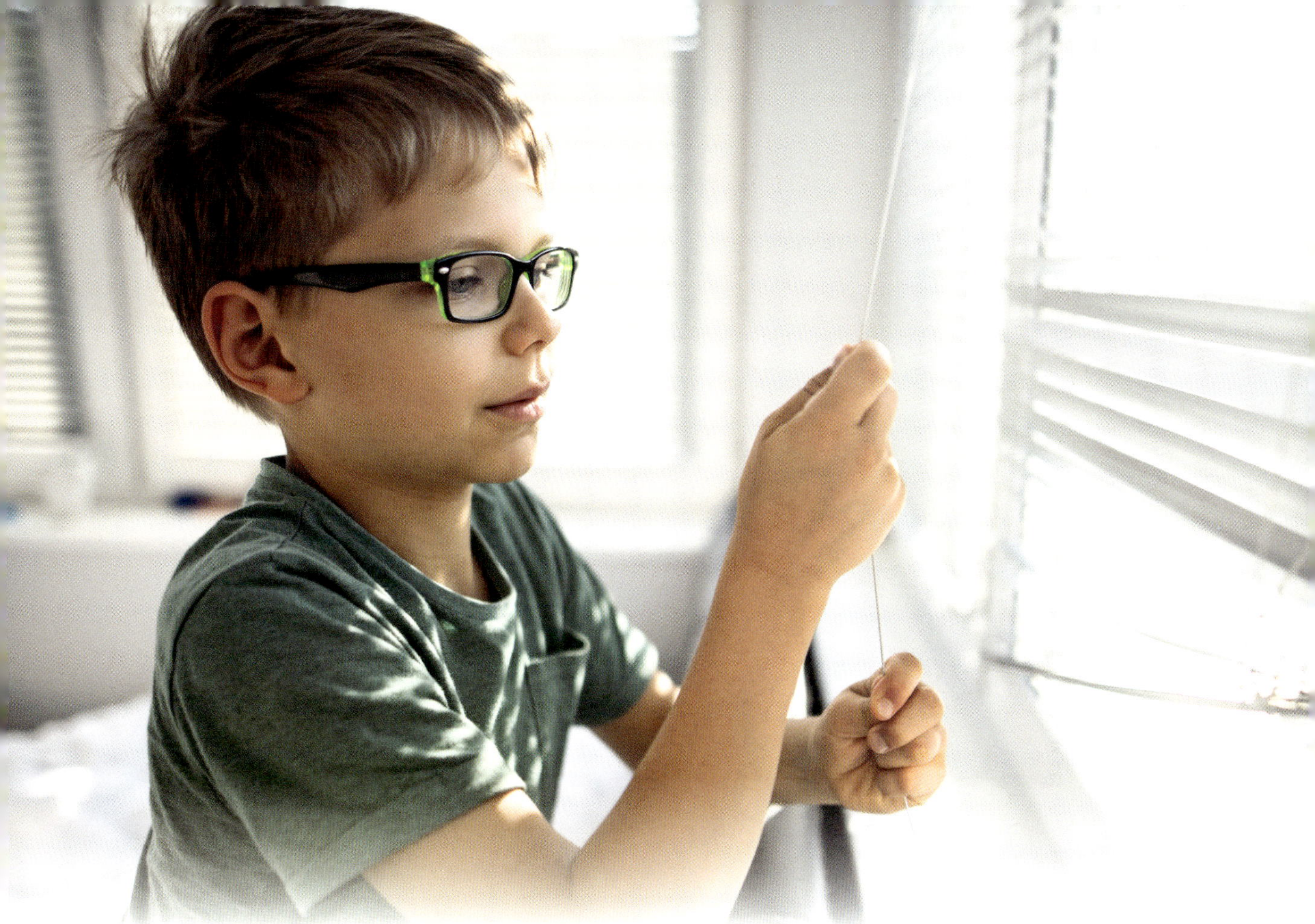

Rest Your Tired Eyes

Your eyes become tired when you read or stare at a computer. This is because you blink more often.

Doctors say to stop working every 20 minutes. Get up, move around. Look out the window. Look at something far away. Ah... don't those trees look calm and peaceful?

The Eyes Have It!

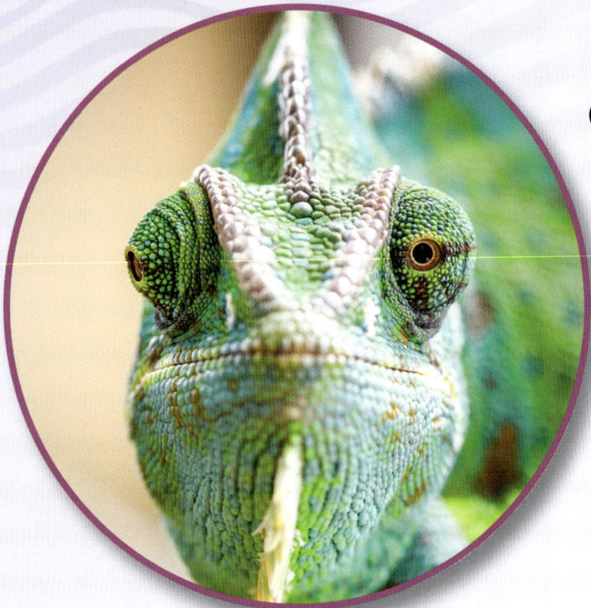

Chameleons can move their eyes in two directions at once.

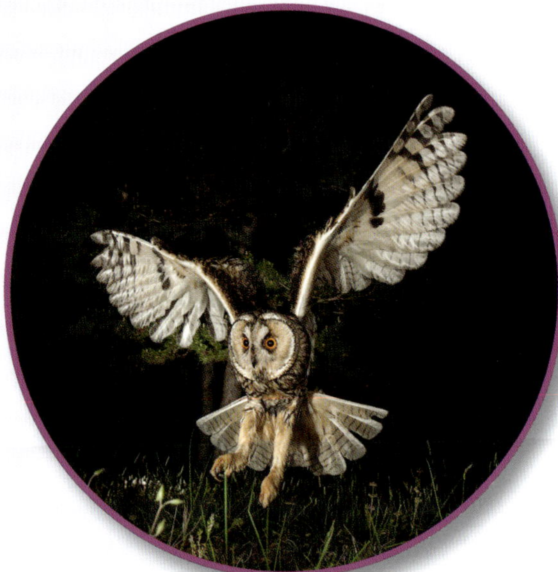

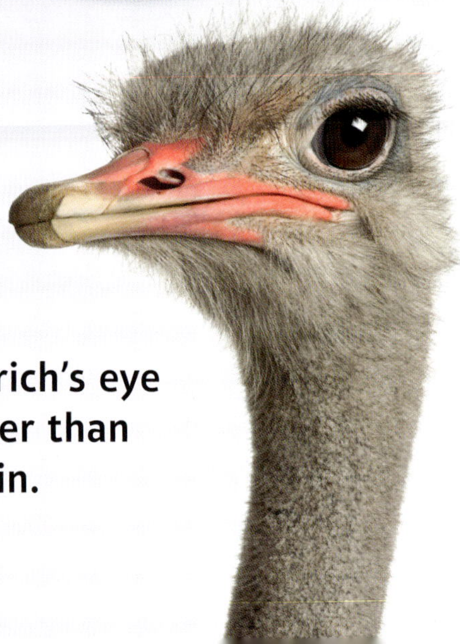

An ostrich's eye is bigger than its brain.

Owls cannot see much close to them. They are excellent seeing things that are far away, even in low light.

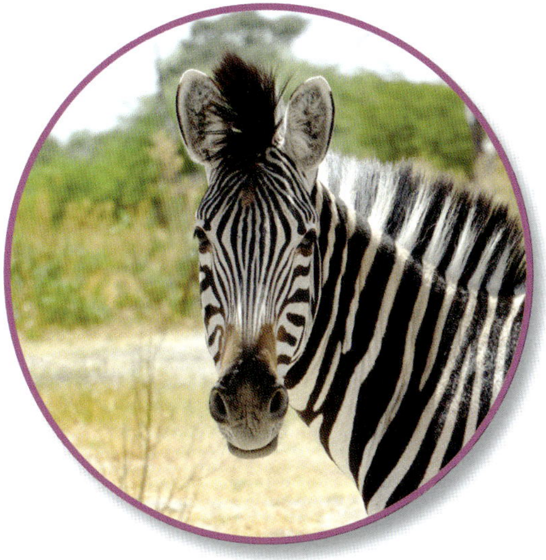

A hawk can see at 20 feet, what we would have to be at three feet to see.

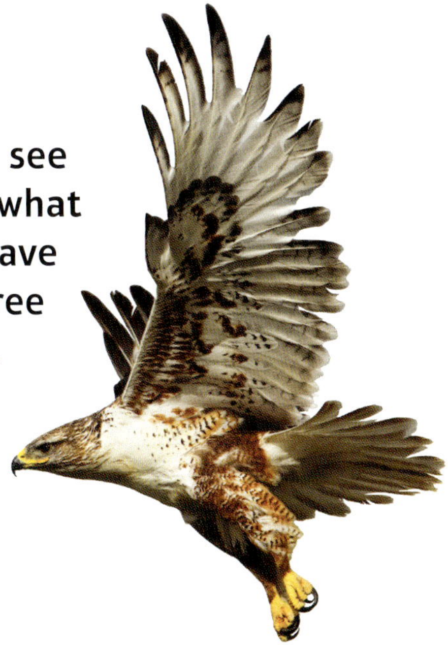

Eyes on horses and zebras point sideways. This gives them great side vision. They are almost able to see behind them. But they can't see right in front of their noses.

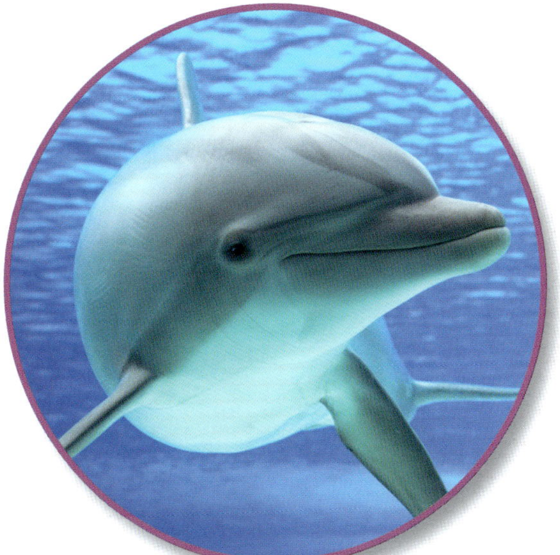

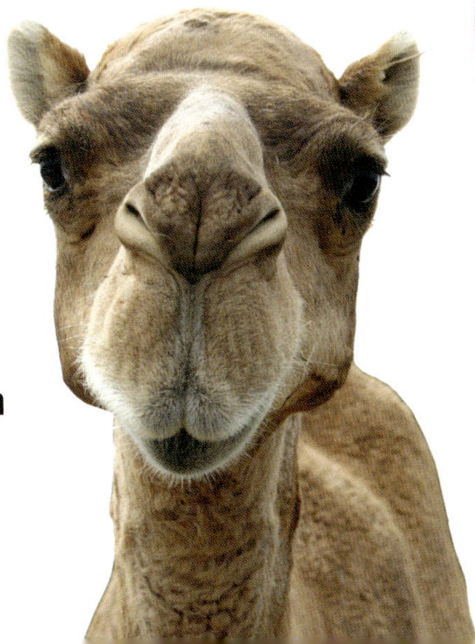

Camels have three eyelids! This protects their eyes from sand blowing in the desert.

Dolphins sleep with one eye open.

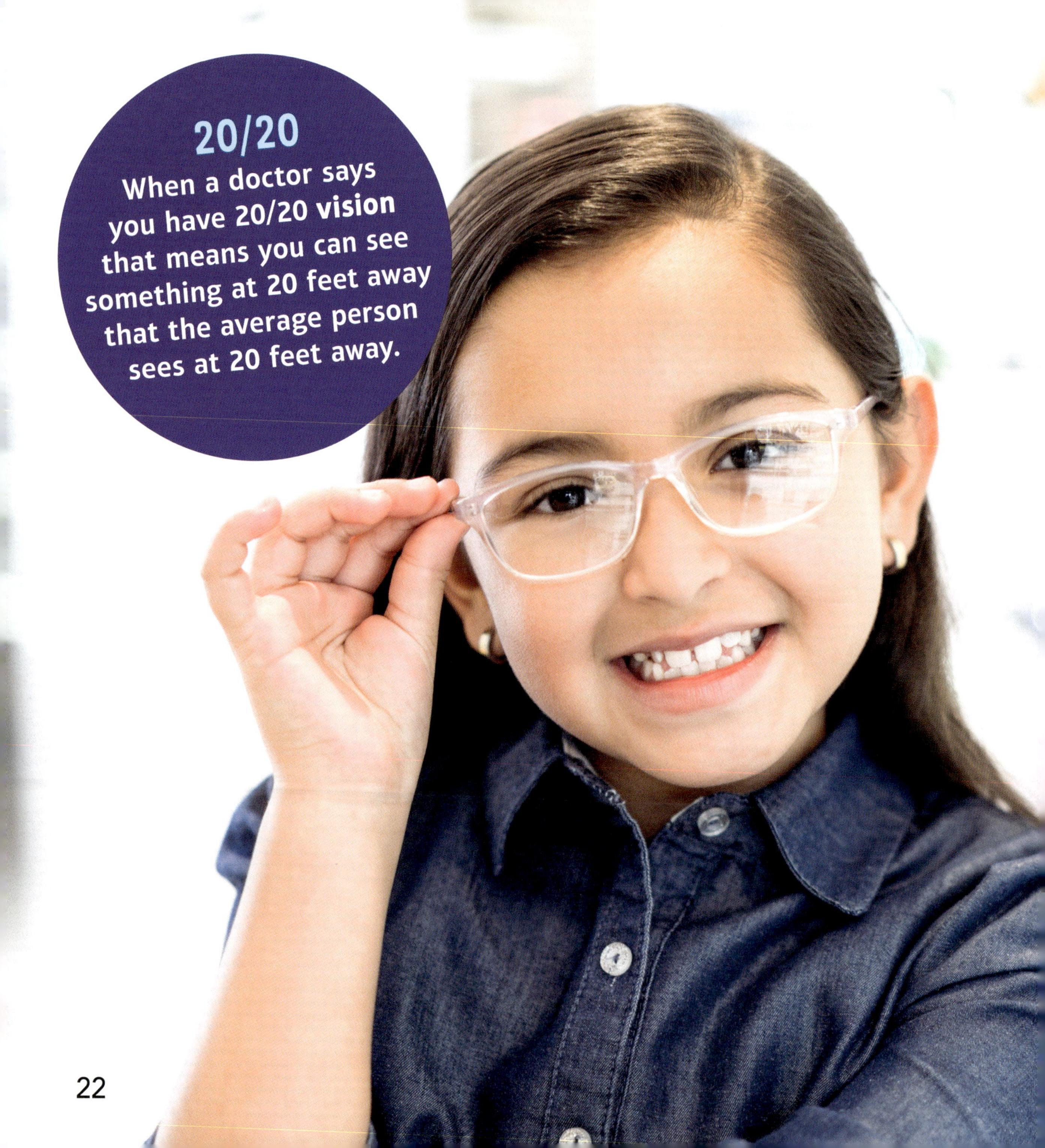

20/20

When a doctor says you have 20/20 **vision** that means you can see something at 20 feet away that the average person sees at 20 feet away.

Words to Know

camera: a device for taking pictures

cornea: thin clear part that covers the eye

eyebrows: help keep dust and sweat out of your eyes.

eyelashes: can catch dust coming and they trap it as your eyelids close.

eyelids: they protect your eyes. Eyelids shut out light so you can sleep. They shut fast if they sense that something is trying to get into your eye. Eyelids blink to keep a watery film over the cornea

image: the "picture" of what one sees

iris: the colored part of the eye

lens: helps the cornea focus light onto the retina

pupil: the dark opening in the center of the eye that lets light in

retina: the part at the back of the eye that sends messages to the brain to create the picture of what we see

tears: your eyes make tears to keep your eyeball clean and wet

vision: being able to see

Learn More at the Library

Check out these books to learn more.

Ballard, Carol. *How Your Eyes Work.* Gareth Stevens, 2011.

Parker, Vic. *Having an Eye Test.* Heinemann-Raintree, 2011.

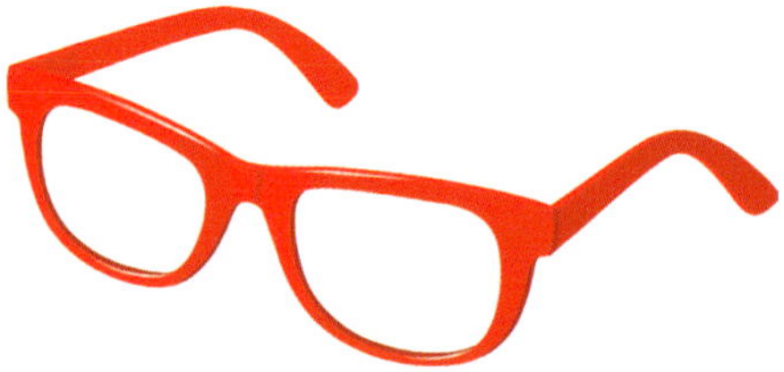

Index

About the Author

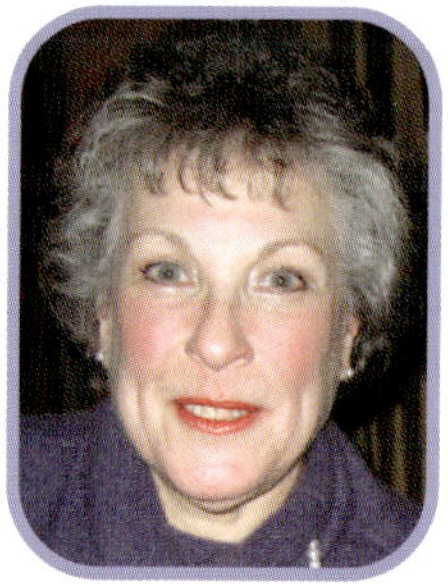

Jeri Cipriano enjoys writing for children of all ages. She loves to learn new things she can share with others.